Mentors & Young Girls Healthy Life

Author: Willeen Williams

Mentors & Girls Healthy Life

MENTORS & Young GIRLS HEALTHY LIFE

&

Living, Eating & Feeling Healthy

Willeen G. Williams

The Alpha Word House Publisher

Copyright ©2017 by Willeen G. Williams

Library of Congress Cataloging in- Publication Data

Washington, D.C

Mentors & Young Girls Healthy Life

by Willeen G. Williams

ISBN- 978-0-9987241-2-6

Printed in the United States of American

Contents

Abstract

It is essential to understand that culture all around the world beliefs are not the same. Some individuals living in different parts of the world will not accept change. There are some people afraid of changes and do not understand the accomplishment that may come out. Some cultures can't adapt to new way of living a healthier life in the community.

It is imperative the mentors get the young girls to conform a virile life. The mentors must have an open line of communication, trust with these young girls. My mission and vision fully express the desires to help young girls look good inside and out to enjoy the upcoming future. The mentor goals to help the individuals to conform more are robust. It is imperative the young girls want to bring about a new change and feel good about transforming and living fit. It is imperative the mentor helps the young girls achieve their goals to finish school and get a college education. It is essential for the individuals to exercise, eating healthier to help fulfill their dreams. Mentors will work with the young girls in a long-term program to help introduce change.

Keywords: Culture, change, transform, learning

Chapter-1 Context Statement

It is essential mentors help the young girls live hearty. There are some individuals struggling with the changes going from one stage of life to another. It is imperative mentors seek the right help for these young girls and help make a difference in their life. It is imperative that young girls have someone they can turn to for help in their puberty stages in life.

"The article focuses on the ways young women and volunteers build empowering connections with sixth -grade girls in the mentoring program" (Brown, 2006, p. 105). There some are young girls that desire the answers to their problems in life. It is important the mentors help empower these ladies from being angry. "The perceived the scale has 14 items assess the degree of life appraised as pressure" (Liang, Tracey, Taylor, & Williams, 2002, p. 279). It is essential these young girls learn how to deal with stress and overcome severe illness.

I will explain to the individuals the mentors will support and will not give up. It is imperative these young girls grow and fulfill a happier life in society. There are programs designed to help young girls redirect and change to healthy living habits. It is imperative the parents get involved and help these students accept change and expectations. It is essential for these individuals to receive the right education, and attend college, and get a good job.

It is important the young girls get involved in the mentor program to enhance encouragement, communication skills, and the knowledge to adapt to life. "There were eight participants self-selected to engage in the weekly club activities with the mentor" (Cayleff, Arteaga, & Dominguez, et.al. 2011, p. 22). It is important for the students learn how to conform to the mentors, and obey the rules. It is essential mentors communicate with the young girls, and allow feedback in the programs. "There were some program conducted at Elmhurst Middle School, sixth-grade girls" (Cheng, Lewis, Stewart, & Malley, 2006, p. 80).

It is important the mentors allow the students to participate and hear the voices, and not be silent. These young girls are suffering from stress, fear and trying to cope with the pain. It is imperative these individuals find peace on the inside and excel in life. "The changes in the community will permit new concepts of leadership and offer a different perspective to alter empowerment" (Hickman, 2010, p. 121).

Chapter-2 Case under Study

"In perspective cases has the profound empowerment to young women to produce a positive development in adolescent females" (Bell, Tracey, Taylor & Williams, 2002, p. 283). It is imperative young girls allow the mentors to help develop a healthy lifestyle. It is imperative the young girls change the old lifestyle to a better way of living. Individuals with low self- esteem will not produce a happy life.

Young girls with high self-esteem will feel good about themselves and live a healthy lifestyle. There are some individuals with low self-esteem will not take pride in dressing, education, and eating habits. It is essential young girls have a sense of peace and encouragement about health, and wellness. "Young women will get depressed changing the gender role in the adulthood into frustration, and stress" (Bell, Tracey, Taylor, & Williams, 2002, p, 271).

It is important young girls receive the proper mentoring during these stages in life to help develop as a mature individual. "Students graduating from college will experience a role shift involves making decisions, education, and careers, financial responsibility" (Liang, Tracey, Taylor, & Williams, 2002, p. 272).

It is imperative young girls leaving from high school to college should have a high level of self- esteem to face the changes in life. It is essential students maintain a healthy life including well- balanced meals and dressing in a professional manner. "Leaders provide special attention, support and encouragement to foster growth and achievement of followers through individualized mentoring and coaching" (Hickman, G., 2010, p. 69). It is imperative for young girls to keep a positive attitude, and enhance confidence, motivation, and communication. There are some challenging moments in life, and inspirational times for young girls trying to find the right direction.

The literature shapes and creates the description to the case. It is about mentoring young girls in the community, school, and help accommodate a healthy living habit. It is imperative young girls have good eating habits, and full balanced meals every day. It is important for young girls to agree with the mentors about healthy living habits.

I care about the well-being of the students living environment. "Servant leaders will play an essential social role in the context of SMO and social institution" (Hickman, 2010, p. 206). It is important individuals learn and comprehend the competence about social and emotion expressions, solving problems and engage healthy relationships. I believe it is necessary for the mentor and the students to continue using good communication skills to help develop growth. "Community support and human society" (Hickman, 2010, p. 135). I believe it is important to have this type of leadership in the community.

It is imperative as a leader to use excellent communication skills, commitment, and trust to help the complete individual assignment. I will represent a clear picture as an entrepreneur for my research project, conform young girls to better healthy living habits. It is imperative for young girls to communicate, and trust the mentors to present change in a professional manner.

"It is imperative trust, cooperation, association, and including foster social goods and services in the community stated by fairness, and well-being" (Hickman, 2010, p. 131). The context of the picture will connect by interacting social media in the community and the reaction of individuals receiving the information. I will help students to apply for the workshop classes to learn more about the program. "Transforming leadership is one or more person engaged in raising another individual on another higher level of motivation and morality" (Hickman, 2010, p. 204, 205).

In organizations, it is imperative leaders coach other individuals to become a director. My desire is to continue serving the community with dedication, trust, and helping young girls, and seeing their beautiful faces reflect in the mirror to a brighter life. It is essential for me to do more research about establishing the retail business online.

The literature is shaping the description of my project helping young girls live healthy and look charming. The research has helped me to bring my picture in a brighter view and establishing vigorous choices for the individuals in the community. I believe it is essential to help people to find the clothing and fashion online without going outside, and right at their fingertips a push of the button.

Chapter 3- Statement of Problem

Over many decades; there have always been problems in the world people continue to face trying to live a healthy lifestyle dealing with stress. It is imperative young girls receive someone to mentor them during the stressful moments. "Personal competence, a moving body is a healthy body, choice and variety for a lifetime, and an emerging sense of gender equity" (Gibbson & Hubert, 2008, p. 167).

Sometimes individuals feel like they are trapped and do not understand the reason for so much stress and low self-esteem the young girl's life. Life is a special gift an individual can behold in their sight. My school will teach young girls how to conform to healthy living habits in everyday life. I will explain the meaning of a healthy life to my students, and that it is the correct way a person lives. It is imperative my students understand their attitude and values it just like a mirror it will reflect back to what they see.

Mentors here in my organization will present a healthy lifestyle to the students and making the right choices, and keeping balance. "It is more 27% say they have experienced stress during the school year, and it has the negative effect on their lives" (Jayson, 2014, p.1). There are overwhelming issues young girls are facing every day in school and even in the community.

My overall goal in the school is to teach young girls to conform and excel in every opportunity in life. There are some young girls from other countries not taught about being healthy. The robust lifestyle of being completely fit is the biggest problem young girls are facing and it is hard to conform to new changes. It is imperative to direct changes, and it is necessary to do things another way to prevent stress. My organization will help the individual to improve health for life, and it is essential to adjust to new changes while trying to put away the old things behind.

It is important young girls learn to respect the rules and the policies of my organization, and will introduce the procedures on the first day of enrollment in the mentoring school. Some young girls had problems with stress changing from another school. It is imperative the person reach out to a friend, cousin or teacher about their situation before it is too late.

Stress will sometimes cause the person to live, and encounter a dangerous lifestyle. "Stress-related eating behavior was more common in girls 43% than boys 15 percent" (Remes & Jaaskelainan, 2014, p. 1). There are some individuals can't understand why the problems taking place in their life, and the cultures are different. Young girls sometimes feel alone and do not know which way to turn for help with their problem. It is important to assistant the person during the stressful moments and help to mentor the student. "Some students have suffered from peer pressure, and needs to change their mindset of the puberty stages that cause the stress to place in their life" (Mc vey, 2007, p. 19). It is imperative the students learn to understand it will take the time to change some of the past habits.

It is imperative the students learn about the school mission statement and help develop education skills, determination, encouragement, and the power to proceed in life. Stress can cause social problems, and the conflicts will lead to anxiety, depression, low self -esteem, poor school performances, and negative thoughts of suicide.

The mentors will establish trust, motivation, and help develop positive change in the student's life. My mentor school has won three years in a row helping young girl conform to change. It is the school's responsibility to maintain the focus on a robust foundation for the student to receive the excellent mentor services. **Young people are** like adults and can experience stress. Stress can come from a variety of things including doing well in school.

It is sometimes it difficult for young people making friendships or managing the expectations from their parents, and the teachers. Too much stress it will create unnecessary difficulty and challenges. Adults are sometimes unaware when their children will sometimes experience the overwhelming feelings of stress in life.

The emotional hints is important in identifying the possible problems, and working with young girls to provide direction to help them achieve in through strenuous times. These are some signs and changes can include such teens may act irritable or moody. Sometimes young girls may withdraw from playing the activities they use to enjoy due to the cause of stress. Young teens, sometimes will complain about school, crying, and acting fearful. It is imperative to watch for the signs of sleeping too much or not eating enough, and sometimes too much food.

Sometimes negative behavior connected to stress, and signs of problems.

It is imperative parents watch these changes, and behaviors in their child. Sometimes, teens will show a signify levels of stress by saying negative things about themselves, and other individuals. Sometimes young girls with a face expression, and it is a sign something wrong with the individual.

It is imperative young teens conform to a healthy living habit. Stress can change a person attitude and eating habits in the home. It is imperative students talk their mentor, parent or another trustworthy adult. Some stress will get a little overwhelming, and it may hard to handle at that particular moment. Parents will sometimes ask too many demands on their child life, and will cause stress to slip in their life. It is essential know the sign of stress in their child face expression. Sometimes young girls in their teen began to promote unhealthy lifestyle by partying and mot eating right foods.

Young teens begin to put things in their body that is not healthy. It is imperative young girls conform, to healthy living habits. Some young teens try to fit in with others at a young age not living a living healthy. It is essential young teens learn to conduct a better life and be proud of themselves. Sometimes young girls do not have confidence in themselves and feel unworthy began to abuse their bodies. It is important that young teens learn they are beautiful inside and out. It is important to take life serious and live a healthy life filled with hope.

Chapter-4 Research Questions

Stress is a problem that individuals battle for decades, and still running rapidly in the land. It is imperative the student recognize the sign of stress, and the effects. These emphases can happen at any event in a person life without warning, and the pressure may get hard to handle. It is the stressor first stage leading the stress to operate at a dangerous point in the student's life.

It is imperative the student understand that stress occurs a little bit at the time, and things will get better in life. It is essential that the individual stay encourage through the rough moment and the pressing days. It is difficult sometimes for the person to see walking through the storm on a rainy day. How does stress related to low self-esteem? There are times stress almost take a complete toll on a person and slip in the midst of their situation. Students sometimes will have problems in school and can't focus in class, and their grades start to drop.

Stress is the leading factor causing the low self-esteem to occur in the individual life, and it is the strenuous blow for the person try to endure. Stress will sometimes cause the student to act suicide, lack of sleep, loneness, avoid social activities with family and friends. There are individual from other cultures do not understand how to deal with stress.

It is essential the individual get back on the right track, and try to restore their life back to a healthy stage of performances. It is important the individual get involve with school activities, and social events, and their life filled with pleasure. Stress is known to affect a person health and the family income. Low self- esteem will cause a negative reaction in the person life, and changing the lives of others. I will extend encouraging word to help the student, and try to get them back on the right track in the classroom,

community, and the home.

Chapter – 5 Methods

Stress is a reaction that deals with an individual emotion or the physical body, and it will upset the young teen natural balance. Sometimes young girls will face, and unavoidable issues may happen their life. There are times in a person's life they with face deadlines in classwork, problems with a loved one. It is imperative they pass exams, and others tests, homework.

The Students trying to get ready the holidays with their friends and family can be a stressful moment. Stress is sometimes a factor that always appears in a person life like, noise, traffic, and pain. A Student can sometimes get stress changing classes, and the temperature may feel overbearing to the young teens. It is imperative young children, and parents learn about coping with stress. Lack of sleep will cause stress in the teen's bodies. Sometimes a person can create their stress in life by worrying about things out of their control. It is essential young girl conform to a healthy living habits.

Some students do not understand the full impact about engaging, confident their appearance. There are teens all of the world may be sitting in a classroom feeling lonely, not worthy, and develop low- self – esteem from all the stress in their life. It is imperative for me gather the information needed to introduce the methods in the research paper to help find the solution to the problems.

"Interviews are among the most common methods of data collection and qualitative research to provide the opportunity to social, and cultural world" (Protudjer, Marchessault, kozyrsky, & Becker, 2010, p. 20). It is essential for me to use all three measures of the methods interview, survey, and observation. "We, therefore, collected information about the participants, the physical and social setting, participant background information, and the process of the program" (Warner, Dixon, & Schumann,

2010, p. 33). Young teenage girls need an extraordinary amount professional mentoring services to help deal with stress. Living a healthy lifestyle is an important part of every individual life. I will visit three mentor schools and, it is imperative to interview students, and teachers. I will start my first assessment to see how the young girls coping with stress in the classroom

- My scheduled is prepared for my conference on August 6, 2015, at 8:15 A.M.

- I will speak to seven teachers to obtain all the relevant information on the young girls in the mentor class.
- The meeting will be held in a quiet and safe environment in a conference always from the school. Zone.

- It is imperative the students have prepared questions to ask and concerns about how the program work for mentor students.

- I have scheduled another conference meeting for the pupils and teachers next Tuesday, August 11, 2015, at 9: 00 A. M.

- It is imperative the teachers present their input and a situation.

- It is essential the mentor in the school continue to carry themselves as good role models.

My second interview is New Press Middle School to present another method to a group of students. I will offer the same method to another young girl in the classroom. Sometimes students will have a different attitude when they are not around their parent. There are some young will say things without a moment notice, and their personal view of the situation. It is essential for young teens to learn about healthy living habits and the benefits of being made complete.

- The parents must sign a permission form, and it will allow me to assessment on their child, and do the interview for all thirty young girls in the community.
- It is imperative I will explain to the parents and students about the consent form and their confidentiality rights.

- The parents will have the access to the location and time of the conference.

- I will send a letter out to the parents, and a text reminder.

- Students will have the opportunity to ask three questioners each.

- The parents are welcome to see the place location before the meeting.

- It is essential to collect the documents from the interviews at the meeting.

My last method is to observe the mentors in the classrooms, and the communication procedures with the young girls in the three different schools. Communication is an important tool to use in the classroom, and the foundation to build, relationship with the students. It is essential for young teens to listen to mentor in the classroom, and learn about healthier living habits.

"The research was conducted on a convenience sample consisting of 1,515 healthy children aged 6–18 years" (Stankiewicz, Pieszko, & Sliwinska, 2010, p. 12). Young girls are learning to communicate and accept that life is better by living more robust. The literature review it is the profound study of the research. It is identifying, and the articulation, the relationship with the field study.

- I will complete my observation in five days and watch the classes performances

- It was important for me to find the right schools for my observation plans.

- I had monitored the mentor's doing their representation for the class with the young girls.

- My observation started at 9:00 until 11:00 and watched the teacher communication skills with the students.

- I gone to the cafeteria for lunch 11:45 until 12:30 to eat, and look at the different variety food groups prepared for the children.

- I had gone back to do an observation from the classroom 1:00 until 2:15 to see the presentation, and the communication with the mentors and the students conform to a vigorous life.

- My observation is completed and collecting all my documents, and the data has been processed on young girls living a healthier lifestyle.

Chapter 6 – Literature Review

In my literature research is about young teens trying to change to a healthier habit. It is an imperative the discussion trying to get young girls to break bad habits. It is important to attend workshops to learn the proper food a person can eat. It is important to look and feel healthy every day, and the appearances of a person lifestyle might impact the young teen's health. "The 8-month intervention program, entitled Healthy Schools-Healthy Kids, was developed around a comprehensive approach, including multiple components at both the individual and socio-environmental levels" (Mc Vey, 2007, p. 119).

The program had helped some children to establish a healthy lifestyle in the community. "Teachers and parents were encouraged to examine their personal attitudes, and beliefs about food, weight and shape issues including raising awareness" (McVey, 2007, p.119). Healthy nutrition is an important part of a person life. Individuals learning to live a healthy is essential to help maintain the proper weight for the person.

"The literature concerning the level of activity of health promotion in faith communities in Scotland, and the views of the leaders" (Fagan1, Kiger, & Teijlingen, 2011). I will have mentors in my schools to encourage young girls when feeling confused or upset. The mentor school will allow parents to visit their child and, help reinforce change. It is imperative that adults and teens learn better behavior, and communication skills.

My research had allowed me to bestow my knowledge upon these teens to flow and excel. It is a fact that young teen girls all over the world need to be the mentor and live a healthier lifestyle. The literature obtained has helped me to apply and enlighten teens to see change and rewarded. There are some teens living in an unhealthy environment and need changes in their life. It is important for leaders in the community help take action to change to a healthier future.

Children will need to develop a healthier habits, and live in a safe environment. Balance is important for students with the guidance of a mentor and gets in the right program. It is imperative that mentor be that lifeguard to give hope to a child that is in trouble. Children in the studies not showing any changes to a healthier living it may cause stress.

There are some disadvantages for not balancing a healthier lifestyle. When teens get the proper amount of care and attention in life, and it can be a better outcome. It is important young girls to get a mentor to help them and do not be afraid of asking for guidance. I have data to prove that young girls need to conform to a healthier lifestyle, and the importance. My research has indicated that young girls need to do better in their living habits.

"The data illustrated from the Creighton University Osteoporosis Research Center were teaching mothers and daughters the importance of building healthy bone mass" (Lappe, & Stubby, 20020). The teens in another mentor school were given a test about the number of bones in the body. It is imperative that mentors address the purpose of a keeping the bones healthy. The information is important documents about the progress of the young girls, and the public schools will help promote to a prosperous life for the students.

Life has an everlasting effect on the individual complete balance and care. Parents should get involved and help educate themselves, family, and the community. It is essential the adults understand that nutrition is important for the students to get all the information and advised from their mentors. A parent should have the report each week concerning their child well-being and nutrition to help produce stability in life. A parent must understand their young teens are trying to make the new adjustment, and it is difficult from the beginning.

It is imperative for teens and parents to set their goals, and strive to finish it in the proper manner. It is essential for the teens to keep a healthy fit body, and a positive mind. It is imperative young people keep a focus on their help. I know that old ways are sometimes hard to break, and it is an important to stay balanced. Positive living habits is taking control of the mind as an individual and doing the right things in life.

It is imperative that the mentors and parents point out to the teens the benefits of life, and living healthy. There are some parents unable to feed their child the proper food. Living a robust lifestyle is a process that need to continue every day. Young teens must be encouraged from the parents and mentors. The parents are their child first teacher and need their help along the way in life.

Community action is important for every individual to get involved and learn about health and fitness.

It is imperative the parents keep raising awareness about upcoming events to help their child change to the healthier lifestyle. Parents in the surrounding counties it is important to help change other young teen's lifestyle. Parents need the education about their child living free from stress.

It is imperative that parent help develop their child growth. It is essential that mentors and parents gain wisdom and help teach in the community. People that do not understand about good eating healthy it will affect their family. It is imperative parents find out where to go and seek health to live vigorously. It is important the community gets out of the comfort zone and help educated, and help young girls learn to live again with joy. Some communities do not have mentors, and it is imperative to get these programs in every county. As a mentor in my community, it is imperative for me to help make changes.

Young girls need mentors in their school to help them cope with their stress and conform and live healthier.

"One study found that about 40% of short-sleeper adolescents reported waking up tired" (Garaulet, & Ortegan, 2011, p. 1314). It is important for students to get the right amount of sleep to stay healthy. There are some young girls that do not have anyone they can talk to about their problems. It is essential as a mentor to help bridge the gap and turn the negative reaction to a position response in the community.

It is imperative to teach more mentors in the community to conform young girls to live a virile life. It is imperative young girls know that someone cares and is there for them in the community. It is important to let the students know there is no need to fear, and learn to live a life filled with love, peace, and a sound mind. It is important young teens learn to love themselves, and love will cast out all fear. It is essential the parents and the mentors have the wisdom and knowledge to build up the young girl's faith, gain trust, and communication skills.

My research has enlightened me with a border view about change in the schools and the community for teens to conform a healthier life. It is imperative that individual's life filled with love and peace. Young teens in other communities need to learn about living a healthier lifestyle and enhance growth. The public should have a volunteer on the street corner, rural areas, and urban areas, and help promote healthier children.

Mentors are special people lending a helping hand to help save a child life. Youth suffering from bad behavior will cause other issues to take place in the person life. Education is important for all the future generation to maintain a positive outlook and try to find the path to travel, and live life to the fullness. Young teens living healthy will produce more quality work in the classroom, and someday in the job market. It is imperative for the young teen to strive for the best in life, and live in a healthy community.

It is easier to close the gap with the lack of knowledge, and the teens get on the right road to healthy and success. It is important for individuals to make behavior changes in their everyday life. It is imperative that young teens have the desire to change for the better. It is essential for the individuals to get help from the mentor about good nutrient and health. Mentors and parents help their youth to develop the changes and it will take some planning to change, preparation, motivation, maintenance, and sustaining the change. It is imperative the mentor develop a successful program for teens to achieve their goals.

Finding Chapter -7 & Conclusions

I have found in my research ongoing needs of young teens trying to conform to healthier living habits. I have learned that some girls from other countries do not use to conform to healthier to better habits. It has been a deep concern to me in my heart to try and the answer to the problems. I have found in my research there are young girls from different culture had problems trying to change their living habits.

"It is imperative to be successful in the local community as a leadership building on the horizontal, local groups, and the international groups" (Hickman, 2010, p. 137). The young teams needed someone to them to adjust to the new culture. My finding have indicated there has been the problem for years young teen living habits need to change. My finding results has shown young girls had problems focusing in the classroom due to not living a healthy lifestyle. It is essential for young to adapt to new ways of living and getting healthy to even the communicate in the community and the classrooms.

It is important for more schools to be implemented with mentor programs to help young girls change to a healthier living habits. It is imperative young girls learn to respect the mentors trying to help them change old ways. Young teens need mentors to help them to adapt to a new culture. There are more being developed to help young teens to conform to a healthier living.

It is imperative to include a diversity to fit in the community for mentoring young girls. The issue with finding individuals living in unsafe environments has been a shock when these finding was reveal to me, and a change needed to help young girls to live a robust life. "It describes the changes that happen during adolescence and how adults can promote healthy development" (McNeely, & Blanchard, 2009, p. 2). There were issues with parents that lived in unhealthy environments trying to work and not paying attention to health and warfare of their child needs, and conform to a healthy lifestyle.

It is imperative the families get the right care to help their child to live more vigorous. It is essential for young girls to adapt to changes, and excel in the healthier position before transitioning to high school. It is imperative young teens learn to change to a live healthy before it is too late. "However, when too much stress builds up, you may encounter many physical and emotional health problems" (Hopkins, 2006, p. 2).

It is essential for the student to have qualified mentors to help them to grow and live a flourishing life. It is imperative for students to get enrolled in schools with a mentor to provide professional skills in the healthy lifestyle, and education. It is imperative to find the solution, and try to resolve the problem with the hands of mentors, parents, community leaders, and teachers. My finding is using the interview has open and closer view of the issue that young girls face in the classroom and the community.

I found it was helpful to sit in the classroom watching the teachers and the students communicate. I believe the results of the finding in the case study is good and understood a better perspective about your teen girls conform to healthier living habits.

I believe the interview was a more affected tool used in trying to solve the problem. My interviews procedures will permit me to communicate with directors, and other officers to help me with making changes with these problems young girls conform to a healthier lifestyle. I believe the conference it will bring some recommendation to the table, and apply it for the community protection, and connect relationship for a more healthy development in the young teens. In my observation were some unhealthy young girls need to conform to healthier living habits. There were mentors, and teachers trained to help young girls promote positive living, developmental growth, and excel in their class performances.

Young girl's life matters it is essential to get adults, and other educators to help bring changes in the community. It is imperative that individuals take these issue serious through the interview, observation can help make changes for young teens in the community. It is imperative these problems addressed to high officers in position to help implement changes.

My research has shown these problems persist for years concerning young girls conform to a healthier living. It is imperative that all culture be included more robust. The early teen years are marked by rapid changes physical, cognitive, and emotional. "Young people also face changing relationships with peers, new demands at school, family tensions, and safety issues in their communities" (McNeedy & Blanchard,2009, 38). These are challenges issues in the community with young girls and trying live a better life.

It is essential girls learning to conform and make progress in school for healthier living in the community. It is imperative these young teens get the help needed to cope with life in the community. Young girls learning to communicate with others are progressing on the right path and getting stronger to a healthier stage of development. Mentors help these young girls live more freely, and someday will transition to another level in life.

It is critical these young teens learn to adapt to new changes in the community and a more advanced lifestyle. My research has allowed me to understand ways to changes the perspective concerning young girls to seek healthy living habits in the community. It is imperative that community leaders help take action to help bring changes, and the aid from the legislature. It is critical parents get involved and the community leaders to promote and enhance the stability in a young girl to conform to a healthier living.

It is important for individuals to stand up and help make a change in their community, and achieve their goals. It is a deep concern to see young girls accomplish their dreams, and step up to live with an empowered mind to success. There are some individuals living with stress every day and can't cope in the classroom or the community.

Young girls were not eating the proper foods, and it will relate to stress and another sickness in their body. It is difficult for young teens to deal with the darkness of stress. Individual's that are suffering from stress is a dangerous illness, and it will not go away on its' own. It is imperative young girls learn the relationship of stress and not eating the right foods. Sometimes students will not eat a balanced meal, and it will sometimes cause the individuals to get stressed. Stress can cause problems to the teen's health, and the no ability to function in the classroom. It is imperative to understand that stress the prime target to some problems in life. Stress can build up from one simple problem to a bigger a matter of minutes.

It is essential for young teen accept the mentor and relate to them about their problem, and help to maintain a healthy life. Sometimes young teens may feel stress from an incident or threat that has happened in their life. Young girls sometimes stress trying to cope with stress, and the person will not have a healthy appetite to eat food already prepare on the table. It is imperative the mentors help young teens to develop a relationship and understand the purpose of the changes getting ready for action.

There are some girls trying to cope with stress, and trying to conform to healthier a lifestyle. Organizational leaders in the program will help the girls with counseling, and answering questions. "Leadership is the cornerstone of a company, and to encourage their employees to reach their goals" (Manning & Curtis, 2009, p.11). Sometimes young girls have a problem with stress, and could lead to other serious issues.

Stress can appear like a big cloud just before it starts to rain, and when it comes it will not stop for a long time. Stress is the dangerous force that can destroy a person life, and it can perform like a bolt lightens and strike the individual without warning. It is essential the person conform to a healthier living habits and is free from low self-esteem.

It is important for a person to engage with positive people and enjoy the flourishing time. I will help the young girls to overcome the negative thoughts in my mentor school, and excel to their dreams. It is essential for the students to stay focus, and do not move backward because it is hard to gain ground again when they lose their position. Mentors have powerful tools, and it will direct the students and help change their culture lifestyle. It is imperative our mentoring school teach professional practice with the young girls to stay motivated, and it will help the individual to understand the purpose.

It is important to enforce changes in the culture environment and enhance the beauty of living more robust. There are goals implemented in the school, and to allow the young girls to reach their level of achievement in the mentoring program. Students are being taught that a healthy living style is important, and it does matter the student need to adapt to the new culture.

It is imperative the individual understand that change does make a difference, and how it can affect everything the person does in the world. The importance of getting the students in my mentoring program to help develop healthier living skills. I will help the students to feel healthy, free to enjoy every moment in life. It is important the mentor and the students have an open line of communication in the organization. Communication is a good foundation for the class to follow, and knowledge gain in the program.

Listening is another key the students must learn to receive the complete understanding in my mentor school, and the expectation. My school is designed to teach the students to achieve their goals and enhance their living habits. I will teach my students how to take charge of being independent, and a brisk existing. "Nutrition education programs are frequently combined with exercise interventions in a community health promotion programs" (Du Plesis, & Incon link, 2011, p. 7).

It is imperative to take pride looking and feeling your best at all times. Students enrolled in my school will continue counseling relating to their health in the program. There are some young teens living in an unhealthy environment and need to conform to a healthier lifestyle. Young girls living healthy, and not living in a stressful situation can do better in school. It is imperative that young teens live a hearty life and adapt to the cultural changes, school, family, and friends. Students can feel internal stress was not eating properly, and experiencing headaches for hunger pains. External relates to something may be going on at home. It is essential young girls to avoid stress, and mentors help young teens to conform to virile life. "These are some stress related factors young girls face that can exemplify" (Marion, 2007, p. 127).

External Sources of Stress

- Overcrowded living conditions

- Moving

- Parents feeling stress

- Divorce

- Poverty

- Joint custody arrangements

- Lots of background anger in the family

- Going to a new school, and leaving the old school

- DIP Classroom

- Feeling child abuse or neglect

- Developmentally inappropriate guidance

- Loneliness or lack of friends

Chapter 8 Recommendations

It is imperative to introduce first leaders, and mentors in the community to help bring change and young teens live a comfortable life in the community. It is essential parents help their transition in a robust lifestyle. Mentors and parents can interpret a robust life for students to accept change, and express a spirit of joy. It is imperative young girls understand the people that care about their health, and the change.

It is important young teens get the proper amount of sleep each night. Individual's stay up late every night it will cause the student to feel tired, and sluggish in class. It is unhealthy for young teens to continue with the lack of sleep and unable to function the classroom. I will recommend the young girls get eight hours every night to maintain a robust lifestyle and perform in a professional manner in the class and the community. Individual's that had gotten less sleep it can cause more stress to attack the person body and health.

Eating healthy and resting is essential in everyday life. I would recommend teens eat the right kinds of foods such as a plenty of vegetables to help support young teens, and plenty of iron and minerals for the body maintain the proper support it needs. There are some process foods that because young girls have stress.

It is imperative teens avoid a lot of sweeteners, soft drinks, fried foods and junk food, pork, red meat, chips and chocolate in their diet. It is imperative recommend that young girls reframe these foods to help reduce weight gain, and it will cause stress. "Healthy lifestyles, the findings illustrated that distance running provides a coping mechanism that can contribute towards health, adaptability and stress resistance" (Shipway & Hollway, 2010, p. 272). It is important for teens to do not put a lot of caffeine in their body. I will recommend teens get into a fitness program to help weight their weight control and assistant to reduce stress. It is important for young teens to exercise to stay healthy.

I will recommend young girls to do meditation position to relax their mind and free from loud noise, and free from stress. It is imperative young girls start walking or jogging every day. Young teens can relief stress by exercise in a group or individual, and it will help relief stress. There are other exercising a person can practice deep breathing to help individual to release stress.

The exercise will work for a person trying it three to four times, and until they feel their stress has be relieved. It is imperative that a person recognize the cause of their stress their life, and try manage the situation. It is important individual take the time to rest and live a stress in their life. The individual have the right mindset to reach their goal. It is imperative a person understand each day a new time. It is important young teens get the support from their parents and mentors to change their eating habits to a bigger variety of healthy foods that nutrition to their bodies. Young teens will need their mentors to help support the changes in their life.

Teens trying to live a healthy lifestyle can be challenging need the support help manage their progress and encouragement. It is important to young girls conform to healthy living every day. It is essential that young teen change those bad habits into a good healthy lifestyle. Young girls will learn to enjoy eating healthy, and once it is the beginning to be a routine practice daily.

There are some young teens engage an unhealthy lifestyle drinking and parties unhealthy living to can destroy their bodies for life. It is important for young teen's first want to make changes and make it a part of their life. It is imperative mentor help encourage young teens, first to love themselves and focus that their life filled with joy, hope, and dreams. It is imperative for young girls to conform they must be willing to change the old habits, and the desire to change a healthy lifestyle. I will recommend as a mentor at school and online twenty- four -hour support team. I will encourage young girls to believe in themselves and never give up. I will recommend young teens to take control of their health by eating right and exercise.

The importance of eating oat meal, fruits, bread, veg. and no soft drinks

- Oatmeal has important fiber to help you feel full for a long time
- Fiber will help control your blood sugar level, and without allowing energy collapse.
- The fiber in oatmeal helps your digestive system.
- Eating oatmeal will help lower cholesterol.
- Whole grain brown bread.
- Fruits, etc. apples, oranges, banana, and water-melons

Mentoring and support team

- The online support team is imperative through email and chat.

- Planning and setting your goals is important.

- Contact mentor to make sure you are on the right track.

- It is imperative to stay motivated through messages from your mentor.

- It is important to speak with your mentor by a phone conversation, one on one Sky sessions.

Exercise to stay healthy

- Bike riding

- Walking

- Jogging

- Taking stairs instead of the elevator

- Join a fitness class.

Appendices

Mentoring for Christ Program

Mentoring Program Form

Dear Parent/Guardian:

Your child has been chosen to strive in the (Mentoring for Christ) offered through his/her school. In the program, your child will be peer with an adult volunteer mentor that will meet him/her at the school. The volunteer will respond as an adult role model in the organization and the inception of friendship and support. The activities between your child and the mentor will be watched and monitored.

It will be structured by the Program Manager in charge of the relationship organization. The school has deep concern all children should definitely benefit in a positive adult role models in his/her life. We hope that child will strive in the mentoring program. It is guarantee to help to increased academic performance, self-esteem, and emotional development in your child life.

The mentors are volunteers for our program have been completely screened and investigated by (Learning to Achieve Program). We are respecting your role as a parent/guardian and will provide you with every opportunity to meet his/her mentor. It is essential for you to stay engaged in your child development in the program, and the mentor services.

During the process of your child attending the program, his/her teachers will monitor all academic performance. All documentation gathered concerning the consequences, and the relationship of your child's school performance is definitely for the purposes of the evaluation of the program will be kept confidential. My school have caring adult volunteers, and will make an excellent contribution to the quality of education in our school. Please talk to your child desires to participate in the program. If he/she is comfortable, and believe that having a mentor is good tool,

please grant your permission by signing below.

One of my Program Managers will soon communicate

with you about your child's new mentor.

Thank you for your time. We hope this program will serve

a great purpose to everyone associated.

Sincerely,

School Principal

I am giving my permission for my child,

_____, to participate

in the Mentoring for Christ Program at his/her school. I

have read and understand the nature and the rules of the

school's mentoring program attempts, and you have reserve

the right to withdraw your child from the program at any

time. I give permission for my child's school documents to

be released to the Mentoring for Christ Program

Coordinator, and mentor to the knowledge that best support

my child's achievement.

Parent/Guardian Signature Date

Courtesy of, Mentoring for Christ Program.

We hope that you will approve of allowing your child

engage in this exciting program at (Mentoring for Christ

Program).

Please free to call if you have any questions.

Sincerely

Sign Organization Representative

_____

_____

Courtesy: Mentoring for Christ Program

Mentoring for Christ Program

Parents/Guardian/ Permission Form
For a Survey

Date: _____, 2015

Dear Parent/Guardian:

Your child, _____(full name), has

been selected to engage in a program, (Mentoring for

Christ), created by (Williams, Inc.). In this program,

(provide description of who the mentors will be and where

they are coming from). A mentor is a caring adult volunteer

who is willing to give their time helping a young student to

succeed. If your child participates, and the mentors will be

communicating with him/her once a week via e-mail while

your child is connecting with us (Mentoring for Christ).

Important information below

The mentors has been carefully screened and trained.

Young girls and mentors are not allowed to meet face-to-face, on the telephone, or at any other place on the Internet without your sincere permission. It is imperative the meeting must take place under your or our close supervision.

Important information below

It is essential your child will be asked to complete two questionnaires—one before he or she is matched with a mentor, and the second near the end of the program it will help us measure and evaluate the benefits and the progress of the (Mentoring for Christ Program). The student will also be asked to participate in a focus group together with the project, and the evaluators present with other youth in the program.

In both surveys and focus groups, and each child will be asked to tell us about his or her view and knowledge with the computers and the Interne, websites, and his or her experience concerning the mentor. Your child's questionnaire information will always be kept confidential and only viewed by professional evaluators. A report

summarizing, and the broader findings will be used to help

us strengthen (Mentoring for Christ) and shared with others

interested in offering the endowment online mentoring

opportunities to young teens.

We hope that you will approve of having your child
engagement in this exciting program at (Mentoring for
Christ Program).

Please call me. If have any question.

Sincerely,

__Mrs. Williams_____

Signature of Organization Representative

(Mentoring for Christ, Inc.)

Please read and return

____ (Initials of parent/guardian) I grant permission for my

child, (*full name*), to participate in (Mentoring for Christ

Program).and will be matched with the right mentor. I will

agree that all communication between my son or daughter,

and with his or her mentor will be kept confidential. I will

acknowledge that if, my son or daughter violate this

confidentiality he or she may be dismissed from future

participation in the mentor program.

__ (Initials of parent/guardian) I grant permission for my

child, (full name), to take the pre- and post-survey

questionnaires and to engage in the focus groups.

____ (Initials of parent/guardian) I grant permission for my

child, (full name), to be allowed a photographed for the

promotional material, media coverage, and communication

_____

Parent/Guardian Signature   Date

References

Anderson, R, (2000). The spread of the childhood obesity epidemic. *Canadian*

Medical Association Journal. 163, (11), 1461.Retrieved from.

http://www.ncbi.nlm.nih.gov/pmc/articles/PMC80413/.

Baumeister, R., Campbell, J., Krueger, J., Vohs, K., (2003).

Does High Self- Esteem Cause

Better Performances, Interpersonal Success,

Happiness, or Healthier Lifestyle? *.American*

Psychological Society, 4, (1). Retrieved from

https://www.psychologicalscience.org/journals/pspi/

4_1.html

Brown, R. (2006). Mentoring on the borderlands creating Empowering connections between,

adolescent girls and young women volunteers. Human architecture: *Journal of the*

Sociology self-knowledge, 1540-5699. Retrieved from the ProQuest Central database

Cayleff, S. Herron, M., Cormier, C., Wheeler, S.,Arteaga, A., Spain, J. & Dominguez. C. (2011).

Oral history and "girls' Voices": The young women studies club as a site of

empowerment. *Journal of International Women's Studies*, 12 (4). Retrieved from

ProQuest Central database

Cheng, L., Lewis, A. Stewart, A., Malley, J., (2006).

Disciplining "girl talk" The paradox of

empowerment in a feminist mentorship program.

Journal of human behavior in the social

environment, 13, (2). The Haworth Press, Inc.

Retrieved from the

ProQuest Central database.

Du Plessis, K., Incolink, V. (2011). Diet and nutrition: *A*

literature review of factors influencing.

Retrieved from, ProQuest Central database.

Gibbions, S.& Humbert, L., (2008). What are middle

school girls looking for in Physical education? Canadian

Journal of F Education. 31, (1), 167-186. Retrieved from

http://www.csse-

scee.ca/CJE/Articles/FullText/CJE31-1/CJE31-

1gibbons%26humbert.pdf.

Hickman, G. (2010). *Leading Change in Multiple Contexts: Concept and practice in*

organizational, community, political, social, and global change settings. Thousand Oaks,

CA: Sage Publication.

Hopkins, J. (2006). Confronting teens stress. Meeting the

challenges in Baltimore City.

http://www.jhsph.edu/research/centers-and-

institutes/center-for-adolescent-health

Ishikawa, S., Kim, Y., Kang, M., Morgan, D. (2011).

Effects of weight-bearing exercise on Bone

health in girls: A meta-analysis. *Sports Med.* 43, p.

875–892.

Jääskeläinen, A., Nevanperä, N., Remes, J., Rahkonen, F.,

Marjo-Riitta, J., Laitinen, L.

(2010).Stress-related eating, obesity and associated

behavioral traits in adolescents: prospect population

based cohort study. *Public Health Journal*, 14, 321.

Retrieved from

http://www.biomedcentral.com/1471-2458/14/321

Karcher, M., (2006). The study of mentoring in learning
environment): A Randomizes evaluation

of effectiveness of school-base mentoring. 9, 99-
113.Retrieved from

Pro Quest Central database.

Laing, B., Tracy, A., Taylor, C A; Williams, L. (2002).
Mentoring college-age women. A

relational approach. *American Journal of
Community Psychology*, 30 (2), 271-288.

Retrieved from the ProQuest Central database.

Manning, G. & Curtis, K. (2009). *The art of leadership.* (3rd.ed.). McGraw-Hill Irwin, Inc.

New York, N.Y.

Marion, M. (2007). (7th.ed.). *Guidance of young children.* Upper Room Saddle.

New Jersey.

Marquardt, M.J. *Leading with questions. How leaders find the right solutions by knowing what*

to ask. (Revised Update). San Francisco: Jossey-Bass.

Northouse, P. (2013). *Leadership: Theory and Practice.* Thousand Oaks, CA: Sage

Publication, Inc.

Mc Needy, C. & Blanchard, J. (2009). A guide to healthy adolescent development. Retrieved

From, ProQuest Central database.

Protudjer, J., Marchessault, G., Kozyrsky, J., Becker, A. (2010). Perceptions of

healthful eating & physical activity. *Canadian Journal of Dietetic Practice and*

Research, 71, (1). Retrieved from,

ProQuest Central database.

Shipway, R. & Hollway, I. (2010). Running free:
Embracing a healthy lifestyle through distance
running. *Perspectives in Public Health.* 130, (6).
Retrieved from ProQuest Central database.

Sigall, B., & Pabst, M. (2005). Gender literacy:
enhancing female self-concept and

contributing to the prevention of body
dissatisfaction and eating disorders. *Social
Science Information.* 85- 111, (1). Retrieved
from,

ProQuest Central database.

Spencer, R., Liang, B. (2009). ''She gives me a break from
the world'': formal youth

mentoring relationships between adolescent girls
and adult women. *J Primary Prevent,* 30, 109–130.
Retrieved from

ProQuest Central database.

Stankiewicz, M., Pieszko, M., Sliwinska, A.,
Malgorzewicz, S., Wieruck,L.,

Zdrojewski,T., Wyrzkowski, B., Szydlowska, W., (2014). Obesity and diet awareness, among polish childen and adolescent in small town and villages. *Cent Eur J Public Health,* 22(1), 12-16, Retrieved from

ProQuest Central database.

Warner, S., Dixon, M., Schumann, C. (2009). Enhancing girls physical activity & self- image; *a*

case study of the go girl go program. WSPAJ, 18 (1). Retrieved from

ProQuest Central database.

Annotated Bibliography

Anderson, R, (2000). The spread of the childhood obesity epidemic. *Canadian*

medical Association Journal, 163, (11), 1461.Retrieved from,

http://www.ncbi.nlm.nih.gov/pmc/articles/PMC804 13/

"A sedentary lifestyle has been found to be

simply related to a adiposity in children"

(Anderson, 2000). It is essential young get the

proper amounts of sleep to function in the

manner. Living healthy is an important source

to obtain a stress free life. It is imperative the

students receive the proper mentoring and

excel in the program.

Baumeister, R., Campbell, J., Krueger, J., Vohs, K., (2003). Does high self- esteem cause better performances, interpersonal success,

happiness, or healthier lifestyle? .*American*

Psychological Society. 4, (1). Retrieved from

https://www.psychologicalscience.org/journals/pspi/

4_1.htmll

"Low self-esteem involves making a disparaging

or low-worth judgement about the self, yet there is

mounting evidence that people with low self-esteem

are not merely negative about themselves"

(Baumester, Campbell, Kruger, Vohs,2003). It is

imperative individuals seek a healthy lifestyle, and

change their environment.

Brown, R. (2006). Mentorinw on the borderlands creating

empowering connections between

adolescent girls and young women volunteers.

Human architecture: *Journal of the*

sociology self –knowledge, 1540-5699. Retrieved

from ProQuest Central database.

"The article focuses on the ways young women

volunteers build empowering connections with the

sixth- grade girls in the context of a girl

empowerment mentoring program" Brown, 2006, p,

105). It is imperative to help young girls to deal

with pain issues in their life, and the community.

There will be concepts used by leaders and mentor

to help the young conform to a healthier life in the

community.

"The analysis has the focus of the three key

practice, and including resisting role modeling, and

how to talk with the girl (Brown, 2006, p, 105). It

is important these girls learn to communicate, gain

trust and give feedback for the organization.

Communication is an important too; to use mentor

yogirls.it is essential the leaders keep a powerful

connection and bridge the gap of doubtful confusion. Itis imperative to continue workshop in the community to help build strong, and healthy young girls.

The leaders and mentor must have a creative background to assistant the individuals with the struggles in the pathway. It is important when volunteers work with these young girls to understand the true meaning of a mentor. The leaders must be able to follow the rules and respect the individual's rights, and privacy.

Cayleff, S. Herron, M., Cormier, C. Wheeler, S., Arteaga, A., Spain, J. & Dominguez. C. (2011).

Oral history and "girls' voices" The young women's studies club as a site empowerment: *Journal of International Women Studies*, 12 (4). Retrieved from,

ProQuest Central database.

"Programs are designed to help improve the young girl's self-esteem, healthier living habits, and complete high school, college" (Cayleff, & Wheeler, 2011, p. 22). It is important for the young girls to have caring mentors to help guide them in life, and be aware of certain things going in the community.

Some young girls will struggle with issues and do not understand how to cope with the problems. Young girls sometimes will get depressed about a love one, and not able to focus in the class. It is important mentor help the individual to overcome that trying moment in life. Leaders can help the person to get their life back on track, and have a higher level of self-esteem.

Cheng, L., Lewis, A., Stewart, A., Malley, J., (2006). Disciplining "girl talk": The paradox of empowerment in a feminist mentorship program. J

Journal of Human Behavior in the Social

Environment, 13(2). *The Haworth Press, Inc.*

Retrieved from ProQuest Central database.

"In the study, the individuals do not fully

agreeing with the empowerment is designed to help

young girls to live a healthier life in the community.

"There was some evidence of the success of the

program, and the staff subverted the goals, and

empowerment to discipline the girls" (Cheng, &

Stewart, 2006, p, 74). The employees were not

understanding the technics the young girls reach the

goals. It is important the individual properly trained

and attend workshops.

Du Plessis, K., Incolink, V. (2011). Diet and nutrition: *A*

literature review of factors influencing.

Retrieved from, ProQuest Central database.

"Nutrients are consumed through the food that we eat, and through metabolic processes in the digestive system these nutrients are absorbed at a cellular level in the body" (Du Plesis, & Incolink, 2011, p. 1). It is important for young girls to eat the right kinds of foods to maintain a healthy lifestyle. Individual living a robust life will benefit in their health, family and friends.

Fagan1, D. Kiger, A. & Teijlingen, E. (2011). A survey of faith leaders concerning health

promotion and the level of healthy living activities occurring in faith communities in *Scotland. Global Health Promotion.* 17, (4): 15–23. Retrieved from ProQuest Central database.

"There was health programs in the faith ministry to help advocate and support the three mechanisms: self-care, mutual aid to help each other cope, and the creation of healthy environments" (Fang, Kiger & Teijlingen, 2011, p. 16). It is imperative for individuals to help them during these types of issues.

Garaulet.M., Ortega, F., Ruiz, J., Lo´pez, J., Be´ghin, L., Manios, Y., Garcı, D., Plada, M.,

Diethelm, K., Kafatos, A., Molna´r D., Tahan,J., Moreno, L., (2011). Short sleep duration is associated with increased obesity markers in European adolescents: effect of physical activity and dietary habits. *International Journal of Obesity.* 35, 1308–1317.

Retrieved from, ProQuest Central database.

"shorter sleepers showed significantly higher values of BMI, body fat, waist and hip circumferences and fat mass index" Garaulet, Ruiz, Lopez, Beghin, Manios, Y., -Garcı, D., Plada, Diethelm, Kafatos, Molna, Tahan,

Moreno,(2011). It is essential for young teens to get the right amount of sleep, and live a healthy lifestyle. Individual staying up late can cause weight gain.

Gibbisons, S., & Humbert, L., (2008). What are middle school girls looking for in physical   education? *Canadian Journal of F Education 31,* (1), 167-186. Retrieved from

http://www.csse-scee.ca/CJE/Articles/FullText/CJE31-1/CJE31-1-gibbons%26humbert.pdff.

"The personal competence, and moving body is a healthy body, choice and variety for a lifetime, and an emerging sense of gender equity" (Gibson & Humbert, 2008). .It is essential students get involved living free and enjoy life without stress. It is important for individual to take out, and maintain a healthy way of living a carefree life.

Hickman, G. (2010). *Leading Change in Multiple Contexts: Concept and practice in organizational, community, political, social, and*

global change settings. Thousand Oaks,

CA: Sage Publication.

Hopkins, J. (2006). Confronting teens stress. Meeting the

challenges in Baltimore City.

http://www.jhsph.edu/research/centers-and-

institutes/center-for-adolescent-health

"Most teens face stress from puberty, changing

relationships with peers new demands of school,

safety issues in their neighborhoods, and

responsibilities to their families" (Hopkins, 2006, p.

3). These issues young teens faces every day in

schools and large cities. It is important young girls

have a mentor to help aid with the issue in their life.

Ishikawa, S., Kim, Y., Kang, M., Morgan, D. (2011).

Effects of weight-bearing exercise on Bone

      health in girls: A meta-analysis. *Sports Med.* 43, p.

875–892.

      "In recent years, the osteogenic potential of

weight-bearing activities performed by children and

adolescents has received increasing attention and

accumulating evidence suggests that this type of

activity may improve bone health prior to

adulthood" (Ishikawa, Kim, Kang & Morgan). It is

important young conform to a healthier lifestyle to

prevent being overweight. Young teen will develop

health problem when than are overweight, causing

stress, and other issues. It is imperative young girls

conform to a more robust life. It is essential mentors

help teen to change their unhealthy living habits.

Jaasklainen, A., Nevanperg, N., Remes, J., Rahkonen, F.,

Jaana, M. (2014). Stress-related eating,

Obesity, and associated behavioral traits in

adolescents: a prospective population-based cohort

study. *Public Health*, (14), 321.

http://link.springer.com/article/10.1186%2F1471-2458-

14-32.

"Stress-related eating is highly prevalent among

16-year-old girls and is associated with low self –

esteem, and as well as adverse dietary and other

health behaviors among both genders, but

intrauterine conditions are seemingly uninvolved"

(Jaasklainen, Nevanperg, Remes, Rahkonen, &

Jaana, 2014). It is imperative young girls learn to

live a healthy lifestyle, and accepts changes in the

cultures.

Karcher, M., (2006). The study of mentoring in learning

environment: *A Randomizes evaluation*

of effectiveness of school-base mentoring. 9, 99-

113. Retrieved from Pro Quest Central database.

"Participate in a multicomponent school-based
intervention program is run by a youth development
agency, assigned these conditions supportive
services" (Lang, Tracey, & Williams, 2008, p, 99).
It stated that young girls had a better outcome to test
than boys. It was imperative the young people have
received the help from the mentors and progressing
at a higher level in school. "Among school girls,
those mentored reported greater connectedness to
different cultural peer, self-esteem and support from
friends" (Lang, Tracy, & Williams, 2008, p. 99). It
is imperative mentors and leaders continue to help
young people excel in life. There are many young
girls from different cultures in the world suffering
from anxiety attacks, depression, eating disorders,
and obesity are unable to function in school. Young

girls will receive professional help from the mentors and leaders give excellent communication, listening skills for a successful outcome.

Laing, B., Tracy, A., Taylor, C. Williams, L. (2002). Mentoring college-age women: A relational

approach. *American Journal of Community Psychology*, 30 (2), 271-288.Retrieved from the ProQuest Central database.

"The traditional conception of mentoring women and girls was rejected and limited in the program" (Laing, Tracy, Taylor & Williams, 2002, p. 271). It is essential develop programs to help individuals cope with their problems. There was research done again and proven that mentoring does help young girls to improve their environment. Individuals have found ways to release stress, frustration, and angry and function in a healthier lifestyle.

Lypazewski, G., Lappe, J., Stubby, J. (2002) 'Mom & me'

and healthy bones: An innovative

approach to teaching bone health. .*Orthopedic*

Nursing. 21, (2), 35- 42. Retrieved from

ProQuest Central database.

"Poor bone health may cause osteoporosis and

an increase for fracture later in life" (Lypazewski,

Lappe, Stubby, 2002, p.35). It is imperative young

girls learn to conform to a healthier lifestyle, and

prevent poor health in teens in the community.

Manning, G. & Curtis, K. (2009). *The art of leadership.*
(3rd.ed.). McGraw-Hill Irwin, Inc.

New York, N.Y.

"The primary function of leadership is to produce and

movement" (Manning, &

Curtis, 2009, p. 12). It is important leaders

communicate with the staff on a professional level

in the company. It is imperative leaders in the

schools are mentors and other organization to

present change working together to excel and

making a difference in the community.

Marion, M. (2007). (7th.ed.). *Guidance of young children.*
Upper Room Saddle.

New Jersey.

"It is imperative teachers express their knowledge

to stop the impact of stress in young children and to

cope with their problem using strategies" {Marion,

2007, p.170). It is important the mentors and

teacher create a safe environment for students. It is

essential the students express their feelings about

stress.

Marquardt, M.J. (2014). *Leading with questions. How
leaders find the right solutions by*

knowing what to ask. (Revised Update). San
Francisco: Jossey- Bass.

"Leaders who lead with questions will create a

more humane workplace as well as a more

successful business" (Marquardt, 2014, p. 8). It is

essential as leaders to bring change in the

organization, and employees will accept change in

the business.

Northouse, P. (2013). *Leadership: Theory and Practice.*
Thousand Oaks, CA: Sage

Publication, Inc.

"Leadership is a process whereby a person

influence group individuals to achieve their goals"

(Northouse, 2013, p. 5). It is imperative a leader of

a qualified person to help employees to agree with

changes in the company. It is essential leaders

understand the needs of the business. Leaders in the

organization will build a foundation

communication, respect with the employees, and

introduce in the company.

Mc Needy, C. & Blanchard, J. (2009). A guide to healthy

adolescent development. *Bloomberg*

School Public Health.

"Adults can provide accurate information regarding physical development, healthy eating, and the effects of media, society, culture, peers, and family on body image" (MC Needy, 2009, p. 13). Young girls are important and need someone to help mentor them through transition from their teen stages into adulthood. It is imperative that young are taught to love, and care about themselves.

McVey, G., Tweed, S., Blackmore, E. (2007). Healthy schools-healthy kids: A controlled
evaluation of a comprehensive universal eating disorder prevention program
Body Image. (4). 115–136 Retrieved from ProQuest database.

"Repeated measures was revealed that participation in the healthy schools-healthy kids program, and a positive influence reducing the internalization media ideals among male and female students by reducing disordered eating among the students" (MC Vey, 2007) . The program has help young teens to live a healthier life.

Protudjer, J., Marchessault, G., Kozyrsky, J., Becker, A. (2010). Perceptions of

healthful eating & physical activity. *Canadian Journal of Dietetic Practice and Research.* 71, (1) Retrieved from ProQuest Central database.

"Understanding conflicting pressures that influence children's healthful lifestyles may enhance communication about these topics among parents, educators, and children" (Protudjer, Marchessault, Kozyrsky, Becker, 2010, p. 19). It is imperative parents get involved about helping their child to conform to a healthier lifestyle. Young girls can function better in school and at home by eating healthy.

Rush, E., Chhichhia, P., Kilding, A., Plank, L., (2010).

Water turnover in children and young

   Adults. *Eur J .Appl Physiol* 110:1209–1214.

Retrieved from

   ProQuest Central database.

   "water metabolism were obtained in a healthy

   multi-ethnic group in children and adults" (Rush,

   Chhichhia, Kilding, Plank, 2010, p. 1209). It is

   imperative young teens drink the proper amount of

   water every day. There are some foods obtain water

   already added. It is important for young girls to

   drink water to keep from dehydration, and living

   healthy favorable outcome mentoring young girls.

Sigall, B., & Pabst, M. (2005). Gender literacy:
enhancing female self-concept and the

Contribute the prevention of body dissatisfaction and eating disorders. *Social Science Information.* 85- 111, (1). Retrieved from,

ProQuest Central database

"Effecting change in schools and communities is an overwhelming, and mentoring programs established young girls to help understand the important living a hearty life" (Spear.2009, p. 109). "It is important for young girls to conform to a healthier life, and to achieve their goals. It is imperative young girls to seek mentor counseling to help them live a healthier lifestyle.

Spencer, R., Liang, B. (2009). "She gives me a break from the world" formal youth

mentoring relationships between adolescent girls and adult women. *J Primary Prevent,* 30, 109–130. Retrieved from ProQuest Central database.

"Formal mentoring programs have historically tended to match the youth with the same-sex mentors; more recently, mentoring programs

designed specifically young teens have begun

cropping up in response to theories on gender and

adolescent psychological health and development,

(Spear.2009, p. 109). There are young teens need

someone to talk too, and help them through trouble

times.

Stankiewicz, M., Pieszko, M., Sliwinska, A.,
Malgorzewicz, S., Wieruck, L.,

Zdrojewski,T., Wyrzkowski, B., Szydlowska, W., (2014).
Obesity and diet awareness, among polish childen and
adolescent in small town and villages. *Cent Eur J Public
Health,* 22(1), 12-16, Retrieved from

ProQuest Central database.

"The addition to genetic predispositions and

environmental factors, healthy lifestyle education is,

an important for children and adolescents"

(Stankiewiez, Pieszko, Sliwinska, Malgorzewiez,

Wieruck, Zdrojewski, Wyrzkowski, Szydlowska, (2010, p.12). It is imperative young girls continue to get the health needed to live a healthier life and live free from stress. It is essential girls learn to listen and conform to better ways, and feeling satisfied in life.

Warner, S., Dixon, M., Schumann, C. (2009). Enhancing girls physical activity & self- image; *A*

case study of the go girl go program. WSPAJ, 18 (1). Retrieved from

ProQuest Central database.

"Girls sometimes will experience problems with negative self-image, eating disorders, low self-esteem, poor body image, and need some help with their situation" (Warren, 2009, p. 29). It is important mentors help young girls to change bad habits for the healthier lifestyle.

www.ingramcontent.com/pod-product-compliance
Lightning Source LLC
Chambersburg PA
CBHW052055270326
41931CB00012B/2772